Gallbladder Removal Diet

A Beginner's 3-Week Step-by-Step Guide After Gallbladder Surgery, With Curated Recipes

Disclaimer

By reading this disclaimer, you are accepting the terms of the disclaimer in full. If you disagree with this disclaimer, please do not read the guide. The content in this guide is provided for informational and educational purposes only.

This guide is not intended to be a substitute for the original work of this diet plan. At most, this guide is intended to be a beginner's supplement to the original work for this diet plan and never act as a direct substitute. This guide is an overview, review, and commentary on the facts of that diet plan.

All product names, diet plans, or names used in this guide are for identification purposes only and are property of their respective owners. The use of these names does not imply endorsement. All other trademarks cited herein are the property of their respective owners.

None of the information in this guide should be accepted as an independent medical or other professional advice.

The information in the guide has been compiled from various sources that are deemed reliable. It has been analyzed and summarized to the best of the Author's ability, knowledge, and belief. However, the Author cannot guarantee the accuracy and thus should not be held liable for any errors.

You acknowledge and agree that the Author of this guide will not be held liable for any damages, costs, expenses, resulting from the application of the information in this guide, whether directly or indirectly. You acknowledge and agree that you assume all risk and responsibility for any action you undertake in response to the information in this guide.

You acknowledge and agree that by continuing to read this guide, you will (where applicable, appropriate, or necessary) consult a qualified medical professional on this information. The information in this guide is not intended to be any sort of medical advice and should not be used in lieu of any medical advice by a licensed and qualified medical professional.

Always seek the advice of your physician or another qualified health provider with any issues or questions you might have regarding any sort of medical condition. Do not ever disregard any qualified professional medical advice or delay seeking that advice because of anything you have read in this guide.

Table of Contents

Introduction

If you want to live a healthy life even if you've just had your gallbladder removed – then there's good news for you! You can definitely live without a gallbladder and you can maintain a healthy and fit life without it – as long as you stick to a diet.

Gallbladder removal surgery is performed on about one million Americans every year. Since you can live without it – many doctors suggest extraction once it becomes inflamed. Typically, inflammation occurs because of inflammation or the emergence of gallstones.

The medical term for removing the gallbladder is called "cholecystectomy" by the layman term is often enough to describe exactly what happens. If you're reading this – then you should already know that most gallbladder removals are done through laparoscopic techniques. This means there's very little invasion of the body and only a tiny cut. Unsurprisingly, this means that some people only need one night to recover from the surgery before being allowed home.

Physical activity is often limited a few days after the surgery. You may also be told to take certain medication to limit pain and infection post-operation. The advice of the doctor may vary depending on how healthy you are to begin with.

No matter how long you stayed in the hospital after your surgery however – it bears noting that the Gallbladder Removal Diet is a life-long commitment. This guide is designed to help you through those years.

By reading this guide, you should be able to learn the following information:

- What your gallbladder does – and why your diet has to change once it is removed.
- The things you can eat – and how it will help you maintain proper health
- The things you're NOT supposed to eat and what happens if you do eat them.
- Dessert, sweets, grease – how to meet your cravings without ruining your diet.
- The healthy amount of food to eat.
- How to prepare your food after gallbladder removal
- On eating out – it's still possible with gallbladder surgery if you know how to frame your orders correctly

- Going on a weight loss diet without a gallbladder – is it possible?
- Enjoy yourself with food even as you accommodate your health needs!

Chapter 1: The Role of Your Gallbladder

What Does the Gallbladder Do Exactly?

The gallbladder – like the spleen or the appendix – are organs in the body that you can comfortably live without. This doesn't mean they have nothing to do in the body however – it simply means that with the right lifestyle changes, you can eliminate the need for their particular function.

The gallstone is a hollow organ located below the right liver. Its main function is to store and secrete bile or "gall" into the small intestines to help process and digest the fat in the food we eat. This function also means that the body absorbs minerals and nutrients better for proper use.

So – does that mean that you can't absorb minerals and nutrients without a gallbladder? Of course not. The gallbladder is just one of the many organs responsible for this task. Without it, absorption still happens – it's just a tad harder for your body. Going on a Gallbladder Removal Diet essentially makes it easier for your body to function without this organ.

What Is Gallbladder Removal?

The surgical removal of the gallbladder, termed cholecystectomy, is a low-risk medical procedure done to treat patients with gallstones.

> Gallstones are pieces of solid materials that result from the accumulation of cholesterol and bilirubin. In the United States, 80% of the diagnosed cases of gallstones are due to high amounts of cholesterol in the diet. While the remaining percentage is strongly linked to patients with liver diseases such as cirrhosis.

The size of the gallstones may be as small as a sand grain or as big as a golf ball. They often occur in the gallbladder and bile duct. The smaller gallstones can naturally exit the body. However, in more serious cases like pancreas and gallbladder inflammation, cholecystectomy is recommended.

Who Are at Risk?

There are many possible factors linked to the occurrence of gallstones. Some of them are discussed below:

Lifestyle

People who indulge in high-cholesterol, high-fat, and low fiber diets are prone to gallstones. This is highly due to the potential of cholesterol in bile to lump together and form gallstones.

> Obesity is also one of the most common causes of gallstones. According to statistics, approximately 25% of severely obese individuals tested positive for gallstones. The excess fats surrounding the stomach as well as the heightened levels of cholesterol in the bile are considered causal agents of gallstones.

Medical experts also advise against crash diet course because rapid weight loss pushes the liver to produce extra cholesterol (in the bile) which in the long run may accumulate and form gallstones.

Biology
Aside from lifestyle, there are known biological factors that increase the risk of developing gallstones.

Age and gender are known risk factors for gallstones. The risk increases with age. Women are also more likely to experience gallstones than men.

Higher estrogen production in pregnancy, hormone replacement therapy, and birth control program increased cholesterol levels in the body all the while slowing down gallbladder processes.

> Lastly, genetics plays a major role too. Individuals with a family history of gallstones have higher risks of acquiring the disease than individuals with no family history.

Underlying Medical Conditions
People diagnosed with diabetes mellitus and liver cirrhosis should take extra measures to prevent gallstones as they have a higher risk.

Side Effects of Gallbladder Removal

All types of surgery come with possible complications. Gallbladder removal is no exception as it poses post-operations risks and side effects for the patient. Here's what you should expect if you've gone through the surgery.

Pain and Tenderness
This one is fairly obvious as all types of surgery can cause pain and tenderness along the cut area. Pain killers would likely be prescribed if the pain is too much along with an advice of limited movement.

Fat Digestion Difficulty
The body will have a harder time digesting fat – which basically means you'll experience some indigestion problems like bloating and flatulence. The body is getting used to the fact that bile is no longer regulated so your diet will be severely restricted during the first few days. It should loosen up a little as you get used to the present set of circumstances.

Diarrhea or Constipation

One or the other could happen after surgery. Indigestion often leads to diarrhea especially if you eat too much fat post-op. Since there's no bile regulation coming in from the gallbladder, this also means loose stool. The constipation is really a side effect of the anesthesia used during the surgery. Once this wears off – and with enough water consumption – constipation should not be a problem.

Injury to the Intestines.
Although it rarely happens, it is possible for the intestines to be damaged during surgery. If pain occurs beyond a few days after a surgery, immediately consult your doctor.

Fever or Jaundice
These two situations are indicative of an infection or if one of the gallstones was not removed properly. Contact your doctor immediately if you notice any of these.

Chapter 2: Gallbladder Removal Diet

What Is It?

The Gallbladder Removal Diet (GRD) is really the diet you will undertake to make up for the fact that your gallbladder is no longer regulating the bile in your digestive system. With this diet, you're essentially compensating for the loss of the organ by carefully choosing what food items to put in your body.

Note that GRD is not something you go on as you "recover" from the surgery. You need to stick to this diet for as long as you live – after all, there's no way your gallbladder can be put back in your body.

Are There Possible Risks or Side-Effects?

Any change you make in your body, including

your diet, may bring about some noticeable

effects.

A gallbladder removal diet highly requires you to transition to low-fat and high-fiber diets. At the early phase of this dietary transition, symptoms like fatigue, constipation, diarrhea, and indigestion are quite common. Abrupt and forceful transition to GRD from your normal diet may intensify these conditions.

However, these medical conditions must remain mild and short-term. If these symptoms persist, consult with your physician.

Moreover, your mental health could also take a hit. The dietary restrictions can be mentally stressful and depriving for some people. The pressure can also fuel anxiety, stress, and depression. To prevent these situations, take small steps. Allow yourself to adjust comfortably.

Foods to Avoid
So what exactly should you kick out of your diet? Here are some of the things you should definitely avoid:

Dairy Based Products
Dairy is one of those food products that can be tough to digest. Anything dairy-based should be avoided which includes cheese, yogurt, butter, sour cream, ice-cream, milk, whipped cream, some sauces, lard, and by extension – all food items having dairy as one of its ingredients.

You can choose to swap this out with plant-based milk such as coconut milk or almond milk or opt for low-fat versions of food.

Fatty Meat Products
Skip high-fat meat which includes pork, beef, lamb, and steak with fat cuttings. By extension, you want to avoid processed food products originating from any of these animals like bacon, bologna, salami, sausage, ham, and others.

Caffeine
Skip caffeinated products which includes coffee, tea, energy drinks, and soda.
Consuming any of these can promote the production of acid, leading to stomach pains.

Alcohol
It goes without saying that you should also avoid alcohol – both beer and the hard kind.

Processed Food Items

Steer away from processed or ready-to-eat food items such as cookies, cakes, sugary cereals, white bread, and fried food. Packaged items are also packed with additional sugar, salt, and fat which is meant to keep them fresh for longer periods. For you however, this translates to digestion difficulties, causing stomach aches. Another notable problem with this is the fact that there's very little nutrition packed in the food, making it more difficult for the body to absorb necessary minerals.

Foods that Can Help
So what should you be adding to your diet?
Here are the ideal inclusions to your food post-surgery.

Food High in Fiber
Without bile, you'd want to make sure that there's enough fiber in your diet to improve digestion. Fibers helps with elimination and creates a firmer stool – ensuring that you don't suffer from diarrhea. Don't go too fast with fiber however – introduce it slowly to your diet so your body can get used to the addition.

Food that's packed in fiber along with other nutrients include:

- Beans
- Peas
- Lentils
- Potatoes with the skin

- Barley
- Oats
- Whole grain bread
- Raw nuts and seeds
- Fruits and vegetables

Lean Meat

You can still eat meat – but you have to be more careful about the kind of meat you're eating. Specifically, you should choose fish products or poultry since they're low in fat. Salmon and trout are excellent sources of meat and fatty acids which helps with digestion. If you're eating poultry however, make sure you're taking off the skin first. Meat alternatives like tofu and legumes should also works wonders in keeping you healthy.

Healthy and Low Fat Food Items

Eliminating a whole food group is usually not a good idea, which is why doctor still recommend the consumption of fat even after having your gallbladder removed. Note though we're talking about "fat" the nutrient here and not the kind of greasy fat usually attached on top of the meat.

Good fats refer to those you can find in avocado, olive, coconut oil, or nuts. Low-fat versions of favorite food items should also be considered and swapped.

Nutrient Packed Foods

Finally, you want to make sure that you're eating something packed with vitamins and minerals. This is important since the lack of a gallbladder severely limits your ability to absorb nutrients and minerals. By eating food dense in the necessary nutrients, you're increasing the chances of getting them in your body for use.

Excellent food products that are rich in Vitamin A, Vitamin C, fiber, and other nutrients include but are not limited to the following:

- Cabbage
- Broccoli
- Cauliflower
- Brussels sprouts
- Kale
- Tomatoes
- Legumes
- Spinach
- Blueberries
- Blackberries
- Raspberries
- Citrus fruits

Meal Portions and Timing

It is true that a gallbladder removal neither affects your life expectancy nor your day-to-day activities. However, aside from dietary composition, health professionals emphasize the need for meal portions and scheduled adjustments.

Remember that the human body is a complete and well-integrated system. Therefore, taking out an organ, no matter how minor its role is (like the gallbladder), will result in slight changes in bodily functions.

Most of us are accustomed to having three big meals a day, breakfast, lunch, and dinner. However, after a gladder removal procedure, it is best to break these big meals into 4-6 smaller meals. Doctors recommend eating small meals every 2-3 hours. This is to help the liver keep up with digestion while providing you with enough energy and nutrients.

Overeating in one sitting may put a lot of strain on your liver because it has to produce a sufficient amount of bile to aid digestion. At the same time, refrain from doing strenuous physical activities after a meal to prevent indigestion.

Chapter 3: Week 1

Having an overview of the do's and don'ts when it comes to food is just the first step in committing to a Gallbladder Removal Diet. You want to be precise with this in order to sustain good health. Here's what you should know:

Listen to the Doctor

Chances are the doctor gave you a good dietary talk before going home. You need to be mindful of what he said and follow it to the letter. Note that this book is simply your second guide – if you have pre-existing health problems, then chances are your doctor considered them before giving you advice. Hence, if his advice is contrary to this book, follow your doctor.

Do a Clean Sweep and Replace

Take a good look at your fridge first and do a clean sweep by getting rid of all the high-fat content. If you live with others, just devote a little corner of the fridge for your stuff.

After the sweep, it's time to pack up your fridge with the right kind of food. Fortunately, there are online shoppers now – even for groceries. Understand that with a Gallbladder Removal Diet – there is no way you can survive with anything canned or microwavable.

Now, chances are there are food items you consume every day like coffee, chips, or energy drinks. Unless they're low-fat already, it's best to avoid them altogether and start on a clean slate – at least for the first week. Give your body a break and skip these items first. Don't worry, you'll have them reintroduced again but slowly.

Aim for Low-Fat Healing Wounds
Since you're also recovering from the surgery, why not try eating food items that promote healing? Anything that's high in Vitamin D, Vitamin C, Protein, and Calcium can help speed up your recovery process. You can get calcium from low-fat milk, protein from fish, and vitamins from fruits like citrus and berries.

Opt for Simple Food
Unless you have someone preparing your food for you, it's usually a good idea to stick to simple food in the meantime. For example, fruits and vegetables can be your go-to food during the first few days because they require zero preparation and you're 100 percent sure the fat is minimal.

Graze on Food

Do not eat three large meals a day since your body is not used to having no gallbladder just yet. You want to keep your food in small portions and distributed all through the day. For example, five meals in small amounts should work perfectly and give your body enough time to properly digest and absorb the food.

Choose Liquid Meals

It's far from appetizing if you're used to big meals – but liquid meals is best post-surgery. This will give your body time to adjust without straining it with solid food products. Don't worry – you can still introduce vitamins and minerals to your diet – just in liquid form. Green shakes and fruit shakes would be perfect and wonderfully easy to prepare.

Stay Hydrated

Don't forget that water should be a major component of your post-surgery diet. Aim for eight glasses of water each day to aid with digestion – especially if you chose to eat solid food instead of softer or liquid meals. Note that staying hydrated should be a priority for all days post-surgery. This is because with no gall bladder, your organs need all the help they can get to properly break down your food.

Observe Yourself

Pay close attention to your body during the first week – and every day thereafter really. It's best to have some sort of food diary where you can record what you eat and what you feel afterwards. Every person is different so you want to make sure that your body is not rebelling against your food choices. Watch out for diarrhea, constipation, flatulence, stomach cramps, and other signs of discomfort and note them down.

Inform your doctor of these instances every time you visit for a follow-up. This will give you a better idea on how to properly frame your new diet for longevity.

Chapter 4: Week 2

By the second week, you should be feeling back to your old self. This is your transition week as you experiment more on different food items you can eat on the Gallbladder Removal Diet. The first week is really all about recovery – which is why your meal plan is focused towards quick fix food items.

During the second week, you're likely more capable of movement and therefore shopping. It's time to play and experiment with your menu through more adventurous recipes.

Establish a Minimum Fat

A no-fat diet post-op is never a good idea. All minerals are important and with fat, you just want to limit it, not remove it entirely. This is why you can choose food products that are "low-fat" and still stay true to your diet.

But what exactly is low fat? Medically speaking, it's anything that contains less than 3 grams of fat per serving. A healthy person – who has a gallbladder – can eat anywhere from 44 to 78 grams of fat per day. For you however, that number should radically go down.

Make Label Reading a Habit

So how do you know that the food contains less than 3 grams of fat? You look at the label of course. Turn this into a habit – especially since most food products today are mandated to come with labels. If you're buying fresh, make sure to check the fat content online.

Note that when reading labels, you should be mindful of the "per serving" situation. You should read this together with the allowable amount of fat per meal for you. For example, if 100 grams of pasta contains 3 grams of fat – then that fits with the 3-Gram Rule. The question however is – how many grams will you actually eat during the day? If you're eating 500 grams of pasta in one serving, then you're eating 15 grams of fat – which is already a lot!

Invest in Food Measurement Tools

For the above reason, it's a good idea to purchase tools that help you measure exactly how much food you're eating. A small kitchen scale will work wonders and give you a better control on what you're eating. Measuring cups for volume would also be a good addition, allowing you to properly prepare recipes according to your dietary needs.

Find Food Swaps

Make a list of the food items that are part of your routine. For example – chances are you drink coffee every day which is now a staple. Unfortunately, caffeine is not ideal after Gallbladder Removal Surgery. So what do you do? Opt for decaffeinated of course!

Here's a list of food swaps you can try for a low-fat diet:

- Ice cream – sorbet, sherbet, low-fat, or fat-free yogurt
- Whole milk – low fat, skim milk, reduced fat
- Sour cream – plain low-fat yogurt
- Ramen noodles – rice
- Pasta with white sauce – paste with red sauce
- Granola – bran flakes, oatmeal, or crispy rice
- Coldcuts – low-fat coldcuts
- Bacon or sausage – Canadian bacon
- Regular ground beef – extra lean ground beef like ground turkey
- Hot dogs – low-fat hotdogs
- Poultry – poultry without the skin
- Oil-packed tuna – water packed tuna
- Whole eggs – egg whites only
- Baked goods – low-fat versions of the same baked goods
- Nuts – air-popped popcorn

- Butter – jam, honey, or jelly
- Oil – non-stick cooking spray

Chapter 5: Week 3

On the third week – you should be ready to go out! Well, you're probably ready on the second week but the third week is the best time to experiment some more outside your own home.

During the second week, the focus is actually on establishing your diet in your own kitchen. During this time, most of your food are personally prepared so you know exactly how much fat you're getting. On the third week however, things get a bit more interesting.

Eating Out After Gallbladder Removal

Sometimes, the difference between low-fat and fatty food is all about preparation. That's fairly obvious from the list given in a previous Chapter. So if you're eating out – how do you know that you're buying something that's low-fat?

The simple answer to this is – just don't eat out. Obviously, that's not always possible as we all have jobs to do and don't always have the time to cook for ourselves.

So what do you do? Here are some suggestions:

- Look for restaurants that have a low-fat menu. Some food providers now understand the value of catering to special diets so this should not be a problem for you. It's a good idea to pick three favorites and just keep going there for you instant meals. If you're a regular customer, then you can be sure that the staff will remember your food preferences.
- If there are multiple portions available, opt for the smallest one.
- Ask for substitutions. For example, instead of fries, you can opt for salad or grilled vegetables as your side dish
- For any kind of dressing, always ask that it be served on the side instead of being added directly onto the salad. This way, you have complete control over how much you actually add to your food.
- You can ask for butter, cheese, or oil to be taken off the recipe
- Look for the words: steamed, poached, baked, grilled, braised, roasted, boiled, or au jus. These are all cooking methods that employ very little fat in the process.
- Some words on the other hand indicate that food is high-fat. These are: cheese, creamed, fried, hollandaise, sautéed, scalloped, basted, au gratin, or anything that contains butter.

- Condiments like salsa, ketchup, vinegar, lemon, mustard, and horseradish are perfectly fine. On the flipside, stay away from whipped cream, cream cheese, butter, margarine, bacon bits, cream cheese, and white sauce.

International Cuisines

Let's say you're in a restaurant serving Japanese food, French food, or some other international cuisine. What do you do? Here's some guideline for a low-fat order:

- French Restaurant – opt for steamed mussels, French bread, béarnaise sauces, mixed greens, and vinaigrette dressings. Wine-based sauces are also the perfect substitutes for the richer types.
- Chinese – if you're eating Chinese, go for wanton soup or anything boiled, broiled, or steamed. The vegetables combined with steamed rice would be good.
- Mexican – grilled chicken and fish would be great combined with jalapeno peppers and vegetable enchiladas. Ceviche, pico de gallo, and chicken fajitas would also be good options.
- Indian – for Indian restaurants, you want to pick lentil wafers or papadum, curries with vegetables, the tandoori chicken/fish, or anything steamed. The shish kabob would also be a good choice.

- Italian – go for the pasta primavera, Italian ices, and roasted peppers. Always go for red clam sauce or marinara sauce instead of the white type.
- Japanese – go for their sushi and steam vegetables. Broiled chicken and tofu-based fishes would also be perfect.

Buying Pre-packed Food Products

At some point, you might have to buy a microwave meal just for the sake of efficiency. While this is best avoided – having a back-up plan would help make sure you're not ruining your diet. Ideally, microwave meals should contain less than 13 grams of fat per serving.

What about the 3-gram rule? The 3-gram rule refers to ingredients for making a meal. If you're buying a full meal however, anything below 13 grams would be ideal – but not the best. The best would still be something you prepared yourself, but that's not something we can all do.

What About Bile Salt Supplements?

Understand the gallbladder removal doesn't mean your body doesn't produce bile anymore. Bile is still secreted – the gallbladder simply regulates its use. With no gallbladder, the bile flows freely into your system. Hence, there's really no need to use supplements like bile salts or enzymes unless your doctor specifically provides otherwise. You can also ask them if you really want to introduce it to your diet.

What about other supplements? If you don't think you're getting enough in terms of vitamins and minerals, the use of supplements is a good idea. Remember though that no amount of multivitamins can replace a balanced diet.

Additional Tips from the Trusted Medical Experts

1.   Start it light. Physicians and nutritionists advise against diving into GRD right after surgery. According to them, it is best if you stick to liquid or soft foods like white rice, banana, boiled potatoes, and crackers.

2.   Do it gradually. Never force your body by changing your diet abruptly. Advance your regimen step by step. Give it time to adjust to reduce digestive symptoms.

3.　　Cook as much as possible. Most of you enjoy munching raw and crispy vegetables. However, with your gallbladder removed, it is wise that you always cook them before eating. This is to help your system digest the food. Steaming is the most amicable method of cooking to reduce oil consumption.

4.　　Tone down your spices. To further help your digestive system, you may need to decrease your cayenne, curry, and cinnamon flavorings. These spices are quite hard on your stomach, thus a little harder to digest.

5.　　No more fried. With frying out of the picture, it is best if you cook your meals using methods like baking, grilling, roasting, steaming, boiling, or the popular air-frying.

6.　　Take it easy with oils. Use oil when extremely needed. Instead of pouring, make sure to use an oil spray. Wipe off any extra oil (on the pan or on your food) using a paper towel. At the same time, butter, lard, and margarine are highly prohibited under GRD.

7.　　Re-invent your salad dressings. This might be your chance to be the king or queen of your own kitchen. Try out inventing your own salad dressing using healthier options like yogurt, lemon juice, and herbs.

Talk it out. Communicate with your peers and family. A lifestyle change such as GRD is somehow stressful and mentally challenging. So, it is better if you express your worries, stress, and feelings towards the diet. You can also try engaging communities (online or offline) with members under the GRD regimen. You can find consolation as well as new friends who can relate in these forums.

Chapter 6: Recipes You Can Try Out

Roasted Veggies

INGREDIENTS:
- ½ pound turnips
- ½ lb. carrots
- ½ lb. parsnips
- 2 medium-sized shallots, peeled
- ¼ tsp ground black pepper
- 1 tbsps. extra-virgin olive oil
- 6 cloves garlic (with skin on)
- ¾ tsp kosher salt
- 2 tbsps. fresh rosemary needles

DIRECTIONS:

1. Cut the vegetables into smaller portions, approximately bitesize.
2. Place and spread the chopped vegetables evenly on a rimmed baking sheet.
3. Place the vegetables inside the oven and set the temperature to 400°F. Make sure that you pre-heat the oven at 350 °F for at least 25 minutes.
4. Roast the vegetables for 15 minutes or until brown and tender.
5. Toss and roast again for 10-15 minutes.
6. Put the baking pan out and let the vegetables cool down for a little while.
7. Plate and serve.

Spinach and Watercress Salad

INGREDIENTS
- 1 cup watercress, washed and stems removed
- 3 cups baby spinach, washed and stems removed
- 1 medium sliced avocado
- ¼ cup avocado oil
- Salt and Pepper to taste
- 1 tbsp. Mediterranean seasoning

INSTRUCTIONS
1. Wash the spinach and watercress thoroughly under running water.
2. Drain and pat the vegetables dry.
3. Remove the stem and separate the leaves of spinach and watercress.
4. In a large serving plate, combine the leaves of the watercress and the spinach.
5. Cut the avocado in half then remove the pit. Then peel the skin off from each side.
6. Slice the avocadoes into thin strips. Set it aside.
7. Prepare the dressing by combining avocado oil, and Mediterranean seasoning.
8. Arrange the avocado strips on top of the watercress and spinach. Season with salt and pepper.

9. Drizzle with the dressing.

Mixed Vegetables and Lemon Zest

INGREDIENTS:
- 1½ cups broccoli florets
- 1½ cups cauliflower florets
- ¾ cup red bell pepper, diced by 1-inch cuts
- ¾ cup zucchini, diced by 1-inch cuts
- 2 thinly sliced cloves of garlic
- lemon zest (2 teaspoons)
- olive oil (1 tablespoon)
- A pinch of salt
- 1 teaspoon dried and crushed oregano

INSTRUCTIONS:

1. Preheat oven at 425°F for 25 minutes.
2. Combine the garlic and florets of broccoli and cauliflower in a baking pan (15-by-10-inch).
3. Drizzle oil evenly over the vegetables. Season it with salt and oregano.
4. Stir the vegetables to coat them evenly.
5. Place the pan inside the oven and roast for 10 minutes.
6. Add the zucchini and bell pepper to the mix. Toss to combine. Continue roasting for 10 to 15 minutes more until the vegetables turn light brown.
7. Drizzle lemon zest over the vegetables and toss.

Salmon and Asparagus

INGREDIENTS:

- 2 salmon fillets, around 5 ounces each
- 14 ounces potatoes
- 8 asparagus spears, trimmed and halved
- 2 handfuls cherry tomatoes
- 1 handful basil leaves
- 2 tablespoons extra-virgin olive oil
- 1 tablespoon balsamic vinegar

PROCEDURE:

1. Pre-heat oven at 428 °F
2. Slice and arrange the potatoes into a baking dish.
3. Drizzle potatoes with 1 tablespoon extra-virgin olive oil.
4. Roast potatoes for 20 minutes, or until they turn golden brown.
5. Add the asparagus afterward.
6. Allow the vegetables to roast in the oven for another 15 minutes.
7. Then, add the cherry tomatoes and salmon onto the mix of roasted vegetables.
8. Drizzle with balsamic vinegar and the remaining olive oil.
9. Roast for another 10 to 15 minutes, or until salmon is cooked.

10. Throw in a handful of basil leaves before transferring everything in a serving dish.
11. Serve while hot.

Arugula and Mushroom Salad

INGREDIENTS:
- 1 tsb white wine vinegar
- 1 tsb fresh lemon juice
- 2 tsps extra-virgin olive oil
- ¼ tsp kosher salt
- ¼ tsp ground black pepper
- 1 cup of quartered mushroom
- 6 oz baby arugula

INSTRUCTIONS:

1. In a medium-sized bowl, add vinegar, lemon juice, olive oil, salt, and pepper. Whisk until mixed well,
2. In another bowl, combine the mushroom and arugula.
3. Drizzle with the dressing (Step 1). Toss well to evenly coat the vegetables.

Seafood Stew

INGREDIENTS

- 2 tsp extra-virgin olive oil
- 1 cut bulb fennel
- 2 stalks celery, chopped
- 2 cups white wine
- 1 tbsp chopped thyme
- 1 cup chopped shallots
- 6 ounces shrimp
- 6 ounces of sea scallops
- ¼ tsp salt
- 1 cup chopped parsley
- 6 ounces arctic char

INSTRUCTIONS

1. Start by heating a frying pan over the lowest setting in your stove. Put a small amount of oil.
2. Afterward, cook the celery, shallots, and fennel for approximately 6 minutes.
3. Pour the wine, two and a half cups of water, and thyme into the frying pan.
4. Wait for 10 minutes and allow to cook.
5. Once much of the water has evaporated, add in the remaining ingredients, and wait for two minutes before removing from the stove.

Tomato Clams

INSTRUCTIONS

- Canola oil cooking spray
- 1 onion, sliced
- 1 tsp minced garlic, or to taste
- ½ tsp salt
- 3 pounds of clams, in shell, thoroughly scrubbed
- 1 tsp red pepper flakes
- 1 cup white wine
- ½ pound whole-grain linguine, cooked according to package directions
- ½ cup chopped flat-leaf parsley
- 4 cups halved cherry tomatoes

INSTRUCTIONS

1. Heat a large pot with a lid over low heat.
2. Spray with vegetable oil cooking spray and add the onion, garlic, and salt. Cook for 3 minutes, stirring constantly.
3. Add the clams, red pepper flakes, and wine
4. Cover and simmer until the clams open, approximately 7 minutes.
5. Add the pasta, parsley, and tomatoes. Cover and let simmer for an additional 3 minutes. Stir and serve immediately.

———

Baked Flounder

INSTRUCTIONS

- 1-pound flounder fillet
- 1 tbsp extra-virgin olive oil
- ¼ tsp salt
- Freshly ground black pepper to taste
- 1 cup halved red grapes
- 1 cup chopped and toasted almonds
- 2 tbsp. finely chopped parsley
- 1 tbsp lemon juice

INSTRUCTIONS

1. Preheat oven to 375°F. Place fish on a sheet tray and season with 1½ tsp. of olive oil, ⅛ tsp of salt, and freshly ground black pepper.
2. In a bowl, combine the grapes, almonds, parsley, lemon juice, 1½ tsp. of olive oil, ⅛ tsp of salt, and black pepper.
3. Place the fish in the oven and bake for 3 minutes, flip the fish, return to the oven -approximately 3 minutes.
4. Remove from oven and top with grape mixture

Vegan Pesto

INGREDIENTS

- 1 1/2 cups fresh basil
- 1/3 cup olive oil
- 1 cup pine nuts
- 5 cloves garlic
- 1/3 cup nutritional yeast
- 3/4 teaspoon salt
- 1/2 teaspoon black pepper

INSTRUCTIONS

1. Gather the ingredients.
2. Vegan pesto ingredients
3. Combine all ingredients in a food processor until nuts are ground. Pesto should still have texture and not be completely smooth.
4. Add more salt and pepper to taste.
5. Vegan Pesto in a food processor

Spinach and Chickpeas

INGREDIENTS:

- 3 tbsp. extra virgin olive oil
- 1 large onion, thinly sliced
- 4 cloves garlic, minced
- 1 tbsp. grated ginger
- 1/2 container grape tomatoes
- 1 large lemon, zested and freshly juiced
- 1 tsp. crushed red pepper flakes
- 1 large can of chickpeas
- Sea salt to taste

INSTRUCTIONS:
1. Add extra virgin olive oil to a large skillet, add onion, and cook until onion starts to brown (about 5 minutes).
2. Add garlic, ginger, tomatoes, lemon zest, and red pepper flakes. Cook for about 3 to 4 minutes.

Zucchini, Celery Greens Soup

INGREDIENTS:

- 1/2 cup cooked green lentils
- 1 parsnip peeled and finely diced
- 1 onion finely diced
- 2 garlic cloves crushed
- 1 green bell pepper cut into small cubes
- 4 asparagus spears
- 1 small zucchini cut into slices
- 1 small fennel bulb finely diced
- 2 celery stalks finely diced
- 1 small bunch celery greens
- 1 lime juice only
- 2 cups low sodium vegetable broth
- 1 tsp chia seeds to garnish
- Freshly ground black pepper

INSTRUCTIONS

1. In a medium saucepan, water fries the onions and garlic for two minutes
2. Add the celery stalks, fennel, zucchini, bell pepper, and parsnip, together with the vegetable broth.
3. Bring to boil, then simmer on low heat for seven minutes.
4. Add the lentils, asparagus, celery greens, and lime juice, and turn the heat off.

---

5. Serve warm, garnished with chia seeds.

Tahini Salmon

INGREDIENTS:

- ¼ cup tahini
- 3 tbsp. fresh lemon juice
- 1 tsp mashed garlic
- ¼ tsp salt
- ½ cup finely chopped cilantro
- 2 tbsp. roughly chopped toasted walnuts
- 2 tbsp. roughly chopped toasted almonds
- 1 tbsp finely chopped onion
- 1 tsp extra-virgin olive oil
- Pinch of cayenne, or to taste
- Freshly ground black pepper to taste
- One lb. wild salmon skin removed, fresh or frozen

INSTRUCTIONS

1. In a bowl, combine the tahini, 2 tbsp. of lemon juice, 3 tbsp. of water, mashed garlic, and ⅛ tsp of salt; set aside
2. In a separate bowl, combine the cilantro, walnuts, almonds, onion, olive oil, cayenne, black pepper, and ⅛ tsp of salt.
3. Fill the bottom of a steamer with water and bring to a boil.
4. Season fish with 1 tbsp of lemon juice, place on a plate and put it in the top of

the steamer. Cover and cook, taking care to remove while fish is still pink inside, 3 to 4 minutes.
5. Remove the fish from steamer, top with the tahini mixture and then with the cilantro mixture.

Tomato and Basil Soup

INGREDIENTS

- 1 medium sized onion
- 1 clove garlic
- 2 tablespoons olive oil
- 8 cherry tomatoes/3 vine tomatoes
- 14oz/400g can plum tomatoes
- 1 teaspoon dried basil or 5 leaves of fresh basil
- ¼ pint/150ml water
- 1 teaspoon salt pepper

INSTRUCTIONS

1. Chop the onions and tomatoes. Then slice the garlic finely.
2. Sauté onion, tomatoes, garlic, and basil in olive oil.
3. Add the canned tomatoes, salt, and pepper. Cover the pan and let it simmer for 30 minutes on low heat.
4. Mash using either blender or food processor.

Cauliflower and Mushrooms Bake

INGREDIENTS:

- 3 cups cauliflower flowerets
- 1 cup fresh mushroom, chopped
- ½ cup red onion, chopped
- 1/3 cup green onion, chopped
- 2 garlic cloves, finely chopped
- 2 teaspoons apple cider vinegar
- 2 teaspoons lemon juice
- ½ teaspoon salt
- ¼ teaspoon pepper
- 1 tablespoon olive oil

INSTRUCTIONS:

1. Preheat the oven to 350 °F. Grease the baking pan lightly.
2. In the meantime, combine red onion, cauliflower, olive oil, garlic, mix mushroom, apple cider vinegar, lemon juice, salt and pepper in a bowl. Mix well.
3. Pour mixture into the greased baking pan.
4. Place inside the oven and bake for 45 minutes. Stir.
5. When vegetables are golden brown and tender, remove from the oven. Garnish with green onions.

Conclusion

Thank you again for getting this guide.

If you found this guide helpful, please take the time to share your thoughts and post a review. It'd be greatly appreciated!

Thank you and good luck!

Lightning Source UK Ltd.
Milton Keynes UK
UKHW020756211222
414213UK00018B/1121